COPYRIGHT © 2024 BENNY MOBLEY

Disclaimer Notice:

Please not the information contain in this book is for educational, motivational purpose only.

Readers acknowledge that the author is not rendering any legal, medical, or professional advice. Please consult your doctor or a licensed profession before attempting any changes or techniques outlined in this book.

Reading this book, the reader agrees that under no circumstances is the author responsible for any losses, direct or indirect, which my incur.

CONTENTS

PROLOGUE

What I am about to share with you is self-discovery from over thirty years ago. These are eight basic pillars to a simple healthy life; I live by and so can you. Humility delivered me from self-destruction of health, mind, body and spirit and an array of health problems later in life.

I invite you on my journey of resilience, triumph, and clarity to a place of peace, health and refuge.

As with all journeys in life growing up in Houston, Texas was a struggle, when I was younger almost everything we ate was fried, saturated, and trans-fat Created through a process called hydrogenation, where hydrogen is added to vegetable oil, converting it into a solid at room temperature.

This process extends the shelf life and improves the texture of many processed foods. which I didn't know at the time, was the worst fat you want to try and avoid all together.

Saturated fats are found in most of your processed foods and meats, oils, lard and tallow etc., it can raise LDL (bad) cholesterol and increase heart disease and stroke. Cause high blood pressure and many other unhealthy risk factors when eaten long term.

Trans-fats are found in ultra processed foods, such as, cookies, potato chips, crackers, fried foods like french fries and doughnuts, margarine and shortening and many other foods found on the grocery store shelfs.

Which can also raise LDL (bad) cholesterol and increase heart disease and stroke, develop type 2 diabetes, weight gain due to high-calorie content and clogging of arteries over time.

Avoiding these two types of fats as much as possible will safeguard your health over time.

Back to my story, when I was younger, we ate fried chicken, pork chops, steaks, liver, bacon, and eggs all fried in lard or Crisco grease, along with other junk processed foods. We thought this was the only way to eat because everyone else in the neighborhood was doing it. It tasted so good at the time. My identity was rooted in fried foods etc.

Today, these bad habits are instilled in our kids due to poor upbringing by parents who learned from their own parents. This is how unhealthy eating habits begin—whether from the environment or the people we associate with as we grow into adults.

Over the long term, these habits lead to obesity, diseases and illnesses. Instead of addressing the root cause—what we eat that's making us unhealthy—we often turn to so-called experts who prescribe medication, which can have long-term side effects and may continue to harm our health. I don't mean to sound preachy, but the truth shall set you free.

I ate this way up until I got married at the age of 23 to 27 years old, I was still accustomed to eating fried foods, not just fried chicken, fried pork chops, steak, bacon, French fries, you name it almost everything was fried.

Until one day, when I was almost 28 years old, I decided to join a gym to learn how to work out/exercise with weights.

Within a two-year period, I started to look different and started liking what I was seeing.

I would also notice my energy level was not changing, I always felt tired after working out, I didn't know why.

Lol the internet wasn't around back in the early nineties, and I didn't own a home computer at the time, well you guess it I had to read about everything through books, magazines, etc.

One day I was at the grocery store, I saw a bodybuilding magazine on the shelf. It said, optimal nutrition sustained energy and muscle mass growth.

My life was changed completely when I discovered it was my nutrition.
I had to change the way I ate, no more fried foods, or processed foods, sugars.

Of course, I had to break this news to my wife at the time.
I was on a new path of living a healthier life. It took another year to break all the bad eating habits I was accustomed to growing up and adapt to a clean eating lifestyle.

Over the last thirty years or so I have gained an abundance of knowledge and wisdom on how to stay healthy, in a holistic well-being sort of way, mind, body and spirit. I will go in deep detail later in my book.

What I will also acknowledge is that people perish for lack of knowledge.

The technology globe we live on today knowledge is right at our fingertips, all we need to do is do the research on a computer your iPhone or android and study the information and implement it to action.

Another valuable lesson I learned, I had mentors who helped guide me on my journey to get better, without faltering or falling back into my old bad habits of eating the wrong foods or not exercising.

Things change throughout our lives but the need for guidance and motivation always endures.

Small simple changes could have a major impact on our health, appearance and most importantly our life.

Helping people is my passion. Living by example as a trainer, coach, motivational coach, life coach, practicing the same simple principles I learned so long ago, I strive to help others in mind, body and spirit.

Allow me to place some clarity on the eight basic pillars for a simple healthy life. To explain the interconnectedness between the mind, body, emotions, and spirit, so that we may unlock vitality and thrive.

Mindset is everything; it's a person's way of thinking—you become what you think. For example, I used to believe my identity was rooted in eating fried foods, and that's how it was. Growing up in Southeast of Houston, Texas, there was no change in that mindset.

Changing this behavior took action with lots of practice and hard work to think differently.

How many thoughts per day do we run through our brains.

According to science research there are anywhere from 35,000 to 70,000 thoughts a day. That is a lot.

When it comes to mindset control, we must have boundaries.

How many of us have had a talk with ourselves like? What college am going to, who am I going to marry, who are your friends? What kind of car I want to buy and so on.

Negative Self-talk can stop any and all progress from moving forward. I can't do anything right" versus "I need to find ways to manage my time better.

We need to be aware that it's actually happening, it's something we need to change immediately.

It stops us from looking at ourselves as the problem. And it makes the real problem clearer: We keep believing what the voice says. More importantly stop listening.

Stressful thoughts produce the stress response in our bodies. Peaceful thoughts produce the relaxation response.

It is equally important to address negative influences that can hinder your progress. Avoiding a negative mindset and low self-esteem is crucial. Here are four things to avoid:

1.   A toxic environment characterized by violence, drugs, anger, victim mentality, low self-esteem, and negative influences.

2.   Toxic people who exhibit low self-esteem, constant complaining, gossiping, being critical and judgmental, cruelty, and manipulation.

3.   Negative digital content on social media, television, in

movies and news. that promote violence, drugs, anger, and other negative content.

4.   Negative music that perpetuates negative self-talk prevents positive thinking.

A negative mindset can come from childhood experiences, trauma, or personality traits.

Negative thinking can lead to mental health issues such as anxiety, depression, ADHD, schizophrenia, and mood disorders. It can also contribute to problems such as social anxiety, stress, and low self-esteem.

Negative thoughts can cause anxiety and depression. Our attitude is important in how we do things, what we think about, what we say to ourselves, what am I going to eat, the things we watch and the music we listen to.

If we want to achieve the eight basic pillars for a simple healthy life, take baby steps of course.

Mindset control is crucial, and I am here to guide you through to accomplishing the pinnacle of your health and life.

The benefits of mindset control/ or change how we think:

1.   More energy
2.   Lower blood pressure
3.   Less stress
4.   Have better Focus
5.   Corrected diabetes
6.   Fat lose
7.   You'll feel healthier

8.   Improved physical health
9.   Improved self-esteem
10.   Improved mental health and quality of life.

To maintain a positive mindset, consider the following:

1.   Read uplifting books that inspire personal growth and authenticity.

2.   Surround yourself with positive friends who challenge you to be your best and offer support when needed.

3.   Engage in regular exercise, which has been shown to improve mood and overall well-being.

4.   Practice positive self-talk and believe in your abilities to accomplish anything you set your mind to.

5.   Cultivate a sense of gratitude and purpose in your daily life.

Body and Exercise, developed from a strong mind, leads to better posture, helps control your weight, and improves your mental health and mood.

It keeps your thinking, learning, and judgment skills sharp as you age, strengthens your bones and muscles, and reduces your risk of certain cancers, including colon, breast, uterine, and lung cancer.

Engaging in regular physical activity is essential for cultivating a stronger and healthier body over time.

There are a variety of options available such as weightlifting, stretching, breathing techniques, and learning proper form to prevent injury.

I hope you're still with me at this point. It will be well worth it in the end. It does get easier over time with consistency.

Which brings me to another key element to accomplishing the eight basic pillars for a simple healthy life.

•Consistency: Staying committed is vital for long-term success. The eight basic pillars for a simple healthy life will help you to maintain consistency in your efforts, be patient with the process, believe in your abilities, and value the long-term benefits of your actions.

changing all bad habits to good ones by taking one step at a time to create new habits to receive better results.

First of all, let's begin why we struggle with being consistent For the first ten days or so, driven by your motivation to meet your goal, you work on your new passion every single day.

But then you gradually start skipping your practice. A day here. A day there. Before you know it, the gym membership has lapsed, you've given up on your coursework, and your cello is in the closet collecting dust. And the cycle begins all over again.

Why is it hard to be consistent?

1.   It's hard to be consistent because we tend to focus on the outcome more than the process.

2.   Put another way, we're more drawn to the positive feelings

or emotions which I will address next, of outcomes rather than the struggle of the journey.

Most of us quit during the struggle before we can experience the rewards of staying on the course.

Commit to the process you have identified for achieving your goals no matter how you're feeling on any given day.

Start with smaller goals such as waking up 5-10 minutes earlier each day and committing to getting out of bed no matter how you feel, uninspired do it anyway.

Understand that the path to your goals is not straight. Anticipation will happen and you will begin to struggle. setbacks, lack of motivation, unforeseen challenges.

Decide ahead of time what you will do when anticipation shows up.

If you want to be consistent, decide to persevere through the struggle. How do you do that? To quote a certain company, "Just do it!" Stick with the basics, spending enough time mastering the fundamentals so that it becomes easy over time.

To believe you can achieve whatever you put your mind to. FIND JOY IN THE PROCESS and find someone to hold you accountable, a wife, a husband, a very best friend, a coach, a mentor, a trainer.

Emotions: Emotions are physical and mental states brought on by neurophysiological changes, variously associated with thoughts, feelings, behavioral responses, and a degree of pleasure or displeasure.

There is no scientific consensus on a definition. Emotions are often intertwined with mood, temperament, personality, disposition, or creativity.

You're problem thinking what emotions have to do with the eight basic pillars for a simple healthy life. Quite frankly a lot, making changes in our lives can be challenging and can make us unhappy, sad, anger, irritable, then we want to quit the whole process all together even before we started.

Then the excuses sat in I'll do it tomorrow, you know what they say about tomorrow it never comes, before you know it another year or two has pass you by and you're still stuck living an unhealthy life when you promise yourself you wanted to live better for yourself and grandkids etc.

I simplify with you challenge is hard but remember these are basic pillars to get you started with easy to follow and understand steps. Yes, it will be challenging to change your bad habits into good ones.

All things are possible with an open positive mindset.

It was hard for me long ago, struggling to stop eating fried foods, it was my choice to stop all fried foods etc, I am not saying you need to give up all your favorite foods, consider eating them in moderations instead of everyday, maybe once every other week or once a month.

Back to my story of overcoming my fried food habits:

As I struggled with this challenge, but I discovered that there's always a solution to solve every problem. Over a year later, I finally stopped eating fried foods altogether.

My solution was to ask my wife at the time to fry and eat it before I came home from work. Once I smelled it or saw it, I wanted to eat it, so this strategy helped me overcome my bad eating habits all together in moderation.

Discovering the eight fundamental pillars of a healthy life has profoundly impacted my well-being, and it can do the same for you. These principles are straightforward to understand and follow.

The only effort required is your commitment to embrace the challenge and achieve positive results along the way.

I guarantee that you'll experience increased focus, sustained energy, and avoid the crash often associated with consuming sugary foods.

Embrace the journey of life by making informed decisions. Understand your goals and life's purpose; they serve as a guiding star.

These eight basic pillars form the foundation: self-awareness, nutrition, physical activity, rest, stress management, social connections, purpose, and spiritual well-being

.

Remember, every choice you make shapes your health-either positively or negatively.

Navigating life's twists and turns often means resisting the pull of conformity and societal norms

.

In our journey, we will encounter numerous challenges that can veer us away from the crowd, from the status quo.

It's precisely in these moments that our inner strength, willpower, and discipline come into play.

Overcoming the temptation to overindulge with friends was a significant challenge I personally conquered over time.

Overcoming challenges like maintaining a healthy lifestyle while surrounded by old habits and friends can be tough.
It's essential to advocate for your health and make choices that align with your goals.

Consistently making healthy choices, even in social situations, contributes to long-term success. It's about building good habits over time.

Enjoying life doesn't mean depriving yourself entirely. Moderation is crucial. Savor your favorite foods occasionally but avoid overindulging. Balance is key.

Planning ahead helps you stay on track. Whether it's meal prepping, having a healthy snack on hand, or scheduling workouts, planning sets you up for success.

Spirituality is prayer divine connection mediation, starting your day with gratitude is a powerful practice. Acknowledging what you've achieved and expressing thankfulness can set a positive tone for the rest of the day.

Purpose and mindfulness play a significant role in overall well-being.

Having a purpose keeps me going, it's not about what I have achieved in monetary or material things; rather, it's a divine connection of the joy I find in investing in other people each day when I wake up.

Having a heart and mind filled with gratitude gives me energy for the entire day.

As a Christian man, I am confident in my identity.
It's the reason I am writing this book: to reach a broader audience and encourage and motivate people all over the world.

We, living in the western world, have our struggles, doubts, and fears, and sometimes we want to give up.

But I encourage you not to quit or give up. Instead, take control of your struggles, doubts, and fears in a positive way by not dwelling on them.

We all face adversities in life. I used to wonder why these things happened to me.

Now I've learned that there's a lesson in adversity-one that teaches us not to repeat the same mistakes and helps us grow.

Finding your identity and purpose will empower you to thrive and grow every day. The eight basic pillars for a simple, healthy life provide the energy and power you need from the inside out.

Believe that you can achieve and take small steps each day. Don't let your mind wander, thinking that these pillars restrict you from enjoying life.
On the contrary, they are meant to enhance your life, allowing you

to live with better focus and energy.

Reminding me of my journey, giving up fried foods was hard. But now that I look back, it was for a bigger divine purpose.

Trusting the process, rather than focusing solely on the journey itself, will help you understand better as you conquer each task to become healthy, spiritually, financially emotions with self control.

Keep up the positive mindset and remember that every step contributes to your overall progress!

I am a living testimony of this myself. My first book was published when I was sixty.

Remember, Colonel Sanders didn't achieve success with KFC (Kentucky fried chicken) until he was sixty-five years old. Why did he succeed at such an age?

Because he refused to quit. I encourage you to do the same- focus your energy on achieving, not on what you lack at the moment, but what you already have. Keep up a positive mindset and remember that persistence will pay off.

Over the long haul, the eight basic pillars for a simple healthy life require commitment, determination, consistency and discipline.

These pillars emphasize the interconnection between the mind, body, emotions and spirit.

Remember to stay focused on these essential aspects of well-being and you'll continue to thrive!

Before I conclude and give you the eight basic pillars for a simple healthy life. I would like to invite you to connect with me in a one-on-one opportunity to help guide you with coaching, mentoring or training.

While it's possible to pursue health goals independently, doing so may take longer to achieve meaningful progress. I've personally experienced this challenge when trying to go it alone.

Struggling to make consistent progress, I eventually decided to hire a mentor or coach.

Their knowledge, experience, and expertise helped me reach my goals faster. However, it was crucial to implement their teachings through action.

Remember: Knowledge without action won't lead to optimal results."
Feel free to adjust this further or let me know if you need any additional assistance!

Contact: www.betterbodytotalfitness.com/holistic-wellness-class

Email: mobley.benny1@gmail.com

Consult your doctor before engaging in any new program.

Introduction

Eight Basic Pillars to a Simple Healthy life

In a world where our struggles are collective, embracing these eight pillars will improve overall quality of life, releasing endorphins, reducing medications, stress, illness, diseases, increase energy, while focusing on a well-balanced lifestyle.

CHAPTER 1 PRAYER PILLAR 1

Prayer- "The best time to pray may depend on personal preferences and energy level. However, starting your day with prayer in the morning, when you're well-rested after a good night's sleep, can be sufficient.

Begin with 5-10 minutes a day and gradually increase as it becomes easier. Praying in the morning can positively impact your mindset for the day consuming positive energy. Start by expressing gratitude for all you have in life.

Praying can help reduce stress and anxiety by allowing you to express your thoughts and concerns, leading to a sense of relief and peace.

Regular prayer can lead to a more positive outlook on life, improving overall mood and emotional resilience.

Praying helps you develop a deeper connection with your faith and spirituality, strengthening your relationship with a higher power.

It can provide a sense of purpose and meaning in life, guiding your actions and decisions.

This approach fosters happiness and joy, rather than beginning the day with a negative mindset focused on things you dislike or lack. Such negativity can lead to stress, whereas gratitude brings fulfillment and joy."

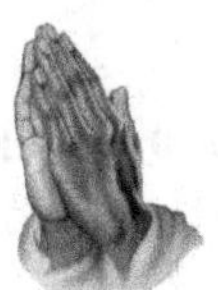

CHAPTER 2 EXERCISE ACTIVITY PILLAR 2

Exercise/Activity: Exercise plays a crucial role in maintaining overall health and well-being.

Incorporating exercise into your daily routines is essential. Consider the following tips:

•Timing: Choose a time that's convenient for you. It could be first thing in the morning before life gets busy or after work.

Discuss with your husband or wife (if you have kids) to find the best time.

•Variety: Whether it's weightlifting, hiking, pickleball, basketball, walking, or any other activity, make it an essential part of your life. Remember, consistency is key!

Regular exercise strengthens the heart, improves circulation, and helps reduce the risk of heart disease and stroke.

Exercising can lower the risk of chronic conditions such as type 2 diabetes, hypertension, and certain cancers.

Longevity: Physical activity has been linked to increased life expectancy and improved quality of life in later years.

The ideal number of days a person should exercise per week depends on their fitness goals, current fitness level, and overall health.

However, general guidelines suggest the following:

For General Health:

Frequency: Aim for at least 3-5 days of exercise per week.

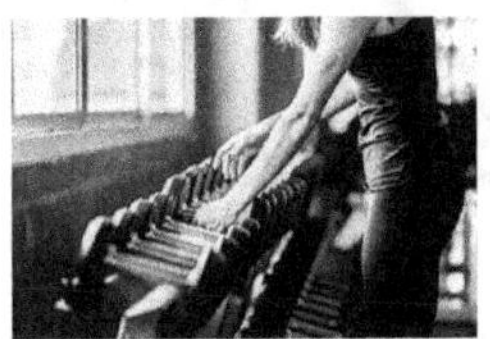

CHAPTER 3 PROTEIN PILLAR 3

Protein- is essential amino acids for overall health and well-being.

It plays a crucial role in rebuilding muscle tissue, maintaining growth, and breaking down and rebuilding tissues throughout our body.

Provides our body with the ability to build strength, sustain collagen, fight off illness, regulate fluid balance, and support various other vital functions.

We need it every day of our lives. Some excellent sources of protein include fish such as cod, halibut, salmon, and albacore tuna, boneless skinless chicken breast, lean ground turkey, eggs, lean ground beef or steak, shrimp, scallops and crabs.

Additionally, plant-based sources like black beans, lentils, and red beans are also great options.

It's beneficial to spread your protein intake throughout the day, consuming protein at each meal every three hours.

This helps support muscle synthesis and keeps you feeling full and satisfied.

Remember to incorporate these protein-rich foods into your holistic lifestyle for optimal well-being!

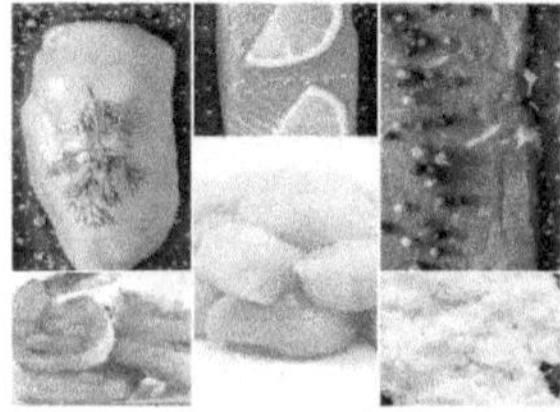

CHAPTER 4 CARBOHYDRATES PILLAR 4

Carbohydrates- Play an essential role in our bodies, and there are two types: complex and simple.

Naturally, we prefer simple carbohydrates over complex, but the simple carbohydrates we should eat in moderation.

Simple carbohydrates, found in refined and processed foods, lack nutritional value and can drain our energy and can cause diabetes.

Complex carbohydrates serve a crucial function in our bodies by providing energy to both our brains and muscles, especially during exercise or any physical activity. Unlike simple carbs (sugars), they are digested more slowly, preventing sudden spikes in blood sugar levels.

Additionally, complex carbs offer essential vitamins and minerals, promote regularity, and support a healthy digestive tract.

To experience sustained energy, consider incorporating foods rich in complex carbohydrates into your diet. Some excellent sources include oatmeal, sweet potatoes, brown rice, quinoa, and wild rice.

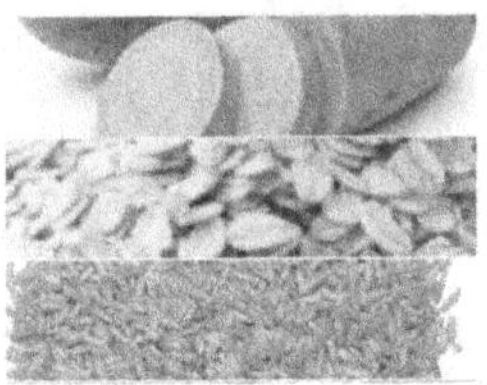

CHAPTER 5 DIETARY FATS PILLAR 5

Dietary Fats- play a crucial role in our bodies, although they are not as essential as getting enough protein and carbohydrates.

However, they remain just as important, especially when following a low-carbohydrate diet.

Good dietary fats provide sustainable energy, protect our organs, support cell growth, regulate cholesterol and blood pressure, and aid in the absorption of vital nutrients.

These fats also help us feel full for longer periods of time and prevent rapid blood sugar spikes, supplying 9 calories per gram.

Additionally, fats serve as structural building blocks in our cells and tissues.

While it's essential to be mindful of fat intake, cutting out all fats can deprive our bodies of what they need most.

There are four main types of fats:
    1. Saturated fats
Found in foods like butter, cheese, and fatty meats.
Consume these in moderation.

    2. Trans fats
Artificially created fats found in processed foods.
Best to avoid this altogether.

    3. Monounsaturated fats
Found in foods like avocados, extra virgin olive oil, and nuts, almonds, walnuts, and macadamia nuts.

These fats are heart-healthy and beneficial.
    4. Polyunsaturated fats
Found in foods like fatty fish, salmon, mackerels, flaxseed oil, chia seeds.

Essential for brain health and overall well-being. Incorporate the good fats-monounsaturated and polyunsaturated fats-into your holistic lifestyle. Consider including avocados, extra virgin olive oil, coconut oil, lean red meat, and other nutritious options.

Avoid as much as you can or eat in moderations:

Avoid Saturated fats and Trans Fats.

Eat more monounsaturated fats and Polyunsaturated fats.

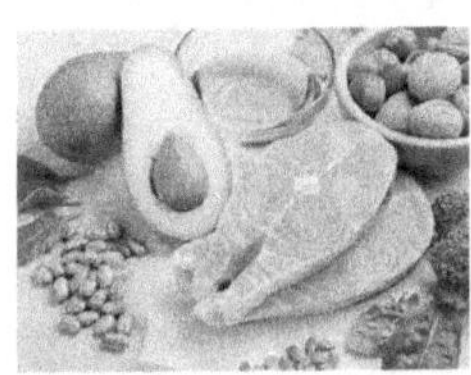

CHAPTER 6 FIBER PILLAR 6

Fiber- Keeps you feeling full longer, which can help with weight management. And its benefits truly are endless.

Help control blood sugar levels.

Aiding in achieving healthy weight.

Lowering cholesterol levels.
Increasing beneficial gut bacteria.
Reduce the risk of certain cancers.

It helps soften your stool, making daily bowel movements easier. Fiber rich foods also provide essential vitamins and minerals.

Some excellent sources of fiber include cruciferous green leafy but not limited to: broccoli, kale, spinach, asparagus, brussels sprouts, green beans, cauliflower, carrots, lettuce, cabbage, moderate fruits, etc.

The general recommendation is that adult women should aim for at least 25 grams of fiber per day, while adult men should aim for at least 38 grams per day.

After the age of 50, this recommendation decreases slightly to 21 grams per day for women and 30 grams per day for men.

Children: The recommended fiber intake for children varies by age. Typically, children should aim for about 14 grams of fiber per 1,000 calories consumed.

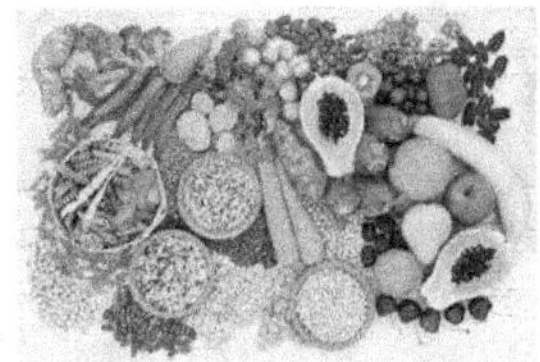

CHAPTER 7 WATER PILLAR 7

Water- The benefits of drinking water every day are essential to our overall health.

Water helps our body temperature regularly from overheating, it maintains a healthy digestion system from becoming constipated, it transports food and nutrients throughout our body.

It keeps our skin healthy and slows down premature wrinkling, delivers oxygen which our body is 60 to 70 percent water.

It lubricates our joints and organs, and adequate hydration ensures the production of salvia and mucus formation, which aids digestion and keeps the mouth, nose and eyes moist.

It also reduces tooth decay when consumed instead of sugary beverages.

The amount of water you should drink each day can vary based on factors such as your age, gender, activity level, climate, and overall health.

The general recommendation is to drink 6 to 8 glasses of water a day, which equates to about 60 to 120 ounces.

This aligns with the daily water intake guidelines to help maintain proper hydration and support overall health.

Keep in mind that individual needs may vary based on factors such as activity level, climate, and overall health. It's essential to listen to your body and drink water regularly throughout the day to stay hydrated.

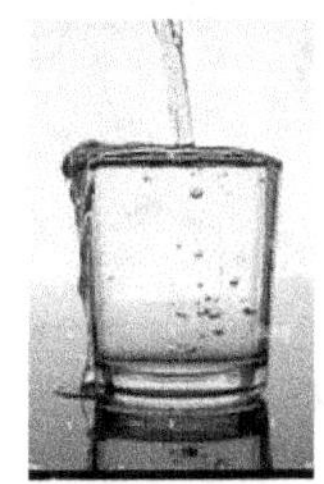

CHAPTER 8 SLEEP PILLAR 8

Sleep- Is essential for our overall well-being and good health.

It helps improve our mood, recharge our mind, body, and spirit after a long day. While we sleep, our body's cells repair and grow, tissues and muscles are restored, and new cells are generated.

During sleep, our heart rate slows down. Insufficient sleep can lead to anxiety and depression.

Adequate sleep helps strengthen your immune system, making you less susceptible to illnesses and infections.

While sleeping, your body repairs and rebuilds muscles, promoting recovery and growth, especially after physical activity.

Sleep helps regulate hormones, including those that control stress, growth, and appetite.

Getting 8 to 10 hours of sleep per night will benefit your overall well-being, and your brain and body will thank you for it.

Remember that our bodies need rest to restore and rebuild after a long day, allowing all the nutrients to function effectively."

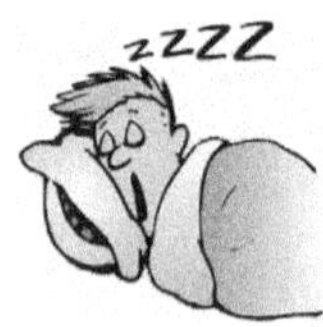

AFTERWARD

These are eight basic pillars I have been living by most of my life and have been healthy by doing so.

Give them a try to live a purpose driven healthy thriving life.

You can still enjoy your favorite foods in moderation once or twice a week instead of everyday and see your health improve over time, eat more whole foods and less processed foods sugars/beverages.

Be determined, committed, consistent and disciplined.

Consult your doctor before starting any dietary plan.

EPILOGUE

As we come to the end of this journey through the Eight Basic Pillars to a Simple Healthy Life, I hope you've found inspiration, guidance, and practical advice to embark on your path to well-being.

Throughout these pages, we've explored the core principles that form the foundation of a balanced and fulfilling life.

We've learned that true health extends beyond physical fitness and nutrition. It encompasses mental clarity, emotional resilience, spiritual grounding, and the ability to cultivate meaningful relationships.

By embracing simplicity and focusing on these fundamental pillars, we can navigate the complexities of modern life with grace and ease.

Reflecting on Your Journey: Take a moment to reflect on your own journey.
Consider the changes you've made, the habits you've adopted, and the insights you've gained. Each step you take towards simplicity and wellness is a testament to your commitment to living a healthier, more vibrant life.

The Power of Consistency: Remember, the key to lasting change lies in consistency. Small, deliberate actions taken daily can lead to significant transformations over time. Embrace the process, be patient with yourself, and celebrate every milestone, no matter how small.

Creating a Ripple Effect: As you continue to integrate these pillars into your life, you have the power to inspire those around you. Share your experiences, support others on their journeys, and create a ripple effect of positivity and wellness. Together, we can build a community that values health, simplicity, and holistic well-being.

A Lifelong Commitment: The pursuit of a simple, healthy life is not a destination but a lifelong commitment. There will be challenges and setbacks, but with the tools and knowledge you've gained, you are well-equipped to navigate them. Trust the process and remain steadfast in your dedication to your well-being.

Final Thoughts: In closing, I want to express my gratitude for joining me on this journey. Your willingness to explore, learn, and grow is a testament to your strength and determination.

May you continue to thrive, guided by the Eight Basic Pillars to a Simple Healthy Life. Remember, simplicity and wellness are within your reach—embrace them wholeheartedly and live your best life.

ACKNOWLEDGEMENT

First and foremost, I want to express my deepest gratitude to God for being my solid foundation and guiding me through every step of this journey.

Without His unwavering love and support, this book would not have been possible. I am forever grateful to my mother, her resilience and wisdom have been a constant source of inspiration, thank you for always being there for me.

To my readers, thank you for embarking on this journey with me. Your curiosity and willingness to explore the eight basic pillars to a healthy simple life have been the driving force behind this book.

I hope the stories and lessons shared within these pages resonate with you and inspire you to navigate your own path to true fulfillment. Lastly, I want to acknowledge everyone who has contributed to the support of this book.
May this book serve as a beacon of hope and a reminder. That true health starts with you. But in staying grounded in our values, faith, and purpose.

Thank you all for your unwavering support and encouragement.

ABOUT THE AUTHOR

Benny Mobley

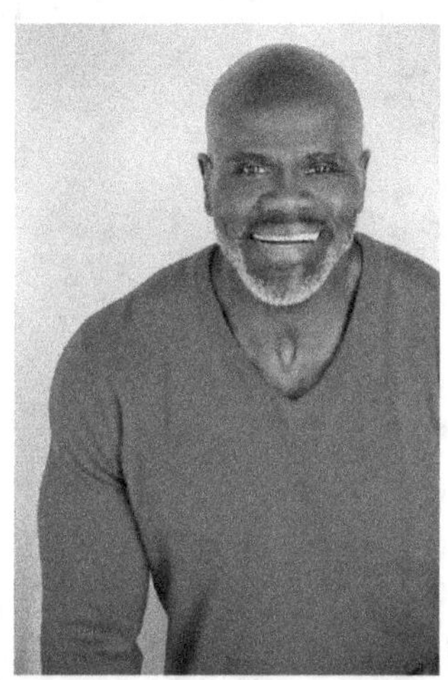

Has been a Trainer, Holistic Motivational Coach and Life Coach for over thirty years. As a Godly Christian man, he is confident in his identity.

He is a former professional natural bodybuilding champion, a professional model, and an author, as well as a co-author. Benny holds a Washington State certificate as a public speaking consultant and owns Better Body Total Fitness.

Where he trains and coaches clients to achieve their optimal health and holistic goals. He continues to strive to help individuals reach the pinnacle of their lives and genuinely cares for their overall well-being.

With a focus on maintaining mental, emotional, and spiritual well-being, he encourages readers to redefine their understanding of a healthy lifestyle and to pursue their goals with integrity and purpose.

Benny continues to inspire and empower others through his work, writing, and community involvement.

When not writing, he enjoys spending time with his two grandsons, training with weights and reading, further enriching his life with balance and joy.

BOOKS BY THIS AUTHOR

Stories Of A Rehabilitated Strongman

by Benny Mobley

Embark on an extraordinary journey of resilience, faith, and transformation with Benny Mobley, a former professional natural bodybuilding champion. In "Stories of a Rehabilitated Strongman," Benny shares his powerful narrative of overcoming life's adversities and emerging stronger and more authentic. Through deeply personal stories, he reveals how he transformed his life through unwavering faith and resilience.

This inspiring book delves into Benny's struggles and triumphs, highlighting the lessons learned along the way. With a focus on holistic health, fitness, and spiritual growth, Benny offers valuable insights and practical guidance for readers seeking to discover their unique gifts, embrace their passions, and live a fulfilling, purpose-driven life.

"Stories of a Rehabilitated Strongman" is a testament to the human spirit's boundless potential and a reminder that, with faith and determination, we can overcome any challenge and find our true calling. Join Benny on this uplifting journey and be inspired to pursue your dreams and live your best life.

Mindset Morning With Gratitude

In a world where adversity is inevitable, Benny Mobley shares his personal journey of overcoming life's toughest challenges with resilience and a grateful heart. "MindSet Morning with Gratitude" is more than just a book; it's a guide to transforming your life by shifting your perspective and embracing the power of gratitude.

Benny's story begins in Houston, Texas, where he grew up in a challenging environment. Despite the obstacles, he discovered that true change comes from within and that gratitude can be a powerful tool for personal growth and fulfillment. Through candid storytelling and valuable life lessons, Benny reveals how he navigated his way from hardship to a life of abundance and fulfillment.

This book offers readers practical steps to develop a morning mindset of gratitude, helping them to see beyond their current circumstances and appreciate the journey. Benny's experiences and insights serve as a beacon of hope, inspiring readers to cultivate a grateful heart and find strength in their struggles.

Whether you're facing financial difficulties, personal loss, or simply seeking a more meaningful life, "MindSet Morning with Gratitude" provides the encouragement and tools you need to transform your mindset and thrive. Join Benny Mobley on this transformative journey and discover the profound impact of living each day with gratitude.

9 798302 021151